Younger Skin Guide for Beginners:

Anti-Aging Natural Skin Care Recipes to Naturally Revitalize, Rejuvenate & Hydrate Your Skin to Look 10 Years Younger

Charlotte Evans

Table Of Contents

Introduction

I want to thank you and congratulate you for purchasing this book!

This book contains proven steps and strategies on how to make skin care products at home that will make you look 10 years younger.

This book will also tell you what causes aging and what the foods to consume to make you look younger

Thanks again for purchasing this book, I hope you enjoy it! Please take some time to stop by and LIKE our Facebook page:

https://www.facebook.com/joypublishing

With gratitude,

Charlotte Evans

Chapter 1 – What Makes the Skin Age?

The skin can age in one of two ways: either internally or intrinsically due to genes that are inherited; or externally or extrinsically due to factors from the environment such as the sun, fumes, smoking, etc.

Starting around age 20, the natural process of internal aging will kick into gear. As a result, the growth of collagen will slow down and your body's elastin will start becoming less flexible. The purpose of collage is to hold your body together and keep skin strong. Elastin is responsible for making your skin return to its original form. Furthermore, as your dead skin cells sluff off, the production of new skin skills will slow down and not replace the old skin as quickly. The results of these processes isn't noticed immediately. Over time, the effects will show themselves and reveal how well or how poorly you cared for your skin.

Below are some of the signs of skin aging:

- Wrinkles

- Fine lines - common around the eyes and mouth

- Transparent and thin skin

- Hollow eye sockets and cheeks

- Skin around the neck and hands becoming less firm

- Itchy and/or dry skin

The speed as to which you age is controlled by your genes. Some people are fortunate to have fantastic genes and look much younger than their biological age. However, there are also individuals that develop the signs of aging in their earlier years, which can be coupled with frustration and despair.

While we can't control our genes, we can control our environment to a greater degree. A huge external factor to the speed of aging is exposure to the sun. Other factors include smoking, gravity, sleeping positions and facial expressions.

Sun exposure can contribute to skin cancer, sun spots, botchy skin complexion and fine wrinkles. Wear adequate sun screen, apply frequently, avoid peak hours of the day, and wear a hat. Anything you can due to protect yourself from the sun will help prevent unnecessary skin aging.

As we make facial expressions, the muscles form grooves and create a memory of that expression. Over time, as your skin loses elasticity, the skin will fail to return to a state of no lines. In return, the grooves will be permanently exposed and show themselves as wrinkles and fine lines. This is common around the eyes since the eyes crinkle when we smile.

The combination of gravity and a loss of skin elasticity will contribute to skin sagging over time.

During sleeping, the way you put your face on the pillow can cause wrinkles and sleep lines to form. Over time, this can imprint on your skin. Sleeping with a silk pillow case is recommended as opposed to cotton.

The chemicals in cigarettes can drastically speed up aging with the skin. Also, consider the frequent position the mouth finds itself in as it's pursed around the cigarette. Similar to the facial expressions factor, fine lines form around the mouth from memory of the muscles used to suck in and blow the cigarette smoke.

Chapter 2 – Foods to Consume for Youthful Skin

Aging can be slowed down with certain foods. Some foods protect the skin from damage brought by the sun. Aside from wearing sunscreen, you should also eat foods that will help you maintain a youthful skin. Such foods will also defend your skin from skin cancer. Examples of foods to consume for youthful and healthy skin are mentioned in this chapter.

Strawberries can help you have youthful skin. Consuming a cup of it daily can give you enough amount of vitamin C. This nutrient will help prevent wrinkles and dry skin due to aging. It also promotes collagen production.

Another fruit to consume more is tomato. It has the carotenoid called lycopene, which evens the skin. According to research that was done on twenty participants, the ones who consumed the highest amount of lycopene possessed even skin. If you have more lycopene, it can safeguard your skin from getting burned. Another study showed that those who were hit with the sun's UV light often possessed nearly 50% less skin reddening once they consumed, aside from their usual diet, two and a half tablespoons tomato paste for ten to twelve weeks.

The study also showed that the ones who took synthetic lycopene or lycopene supplement were not really safeguarded from sunburn. This means supplements will not work the way real food sources would. Lycopene can be found in carrots, guava, pink grapefruit, red peppers and watermelon.

Another food that will make your skin youthful is tofu. It helps in preserving collagen because of its high content of isoflavones. In one study, mice that were given isoflavones and were hit with UV radiation had smoother skin and lesser wrinkles as compared to those that did not consume isoflavones but were exposed to the sun's UV light. Researchers then concluded isoflavones can prevent the breakdown of collagen. Aside from tofu, you can also consume soy-based foods.

Tuna is also another food that will make the skin look younger because it contains so much omega-3 fatty acids. Aside from tuna, sardines and salmon can also make the skin look younger. These types of fish can also protect you from skin cancer because of their eicosapentaenoic acid content which preserves collagen. They also have docosahexaenoic acid which protects you from skin cancer because it decreases inflammatory compounds that stimulate the growth of tumors. It is advisable to consume a couple of servings of these types of fish per week because they are also beneficial to the heart.

Coffee can also make the skin younger, and consuming a cup of it every day may reduce the risk of having skin cancer. According to a study which had more than 93,000 female participants, those who consumed a cup of coffee per day lowered by 10% the risk of having nonmelanoma skin cancer. If they consumed more than this daily, the risk is all the more reduced. The study claims that decaffeinated coffee did not seem to give a similar protection.

Consuming chocolates is said to give acne. Studies show, however, that a link between skin disorders and chocolate does not exist. These studies also say there are some kinds of chocolate that promote good skin. This is because cocoa has epicatechin, a kind of flavonoid which is also found in red wine and tea. According to a study involving 24 females, consuming cocoa that is rich in epicatechin every day for three months improved the texture of the skin. This is because epicatechin increases blood circulation in the skin and enhances the supply of oxygen and nutrients which make the skin healthy and youthful.

Aside from consuming these foods, you can also formulate and use skin care products with kitchen ingredients to ensure that your skin remains young and clean. The rest of the chapters of this book will give you recipes on how to make a facial scrub, cleaner, toner, moisturizer and mask using ingredients found at home.

Chapter 3 – Anti-aging Facial Scrubs

One of the most important parts of an anti-aging skincare regimen is exfoliation. It removes dead skin cells and allows the face to form new ones. If you do not remove these dead skin cells, they will accumulate and turn into darker spots that are referred to as age spots. Exfoliation must be done twice or thrice per week. Many people though do not exfoliate or scrub their faces because the facial scrubs in the market can be very expensive and may have harsh chemicals.

The good news is you can make effective facial scrubs using kitchen ingredients. Not only are they safe, but they are also cost-effective. You will have a clean and youthful skin with these homemade scrubs.

Before using these scrubs, you should first tie your hair back. Take off makeup you have on and wash your face with warm water. For the pores on your face to open, press a warm cloth on your face for a few minutes. You can also use the steam coming from hot water. Apply the facial scrub on your face but make sure not to put some on your eye area. You can also apply the scrub on your neck. Rinse your face using warm water. For maximum exfoliation, you can utilize a sponge, brush or loofah made for the face.

Simple Baking Soda Facial Exfoliator

This facial scrub can be used daily because of its mildness.

Ingredients:

- Two to three tablespoons of baking soda
- Water (tiny amount only)

Procedure:

1. Mix baking soda and enough amount of water to make a paste.
2. Wash your face with warm water.
3. Apply and scrub gently the paste on your face in a circular movement.
4. Rinse with warm water

This facial scrub can be used every day because it is mild.

Simple Cornmeal Facial Exfoliator

This facial scrub can be used after two to three days as it is a bit stronger than the baking soda exfoliator.

Ingredients:

- Two to three tablespoons of cornmeal
- Tiny amount of water

Procedure:

1. Wash your face with warm water.
2. Combine the two ingredients to form a paste.
3. Apply on your face
4. Rinse with warm water

Rose Almond Facial Exfoliator

This facial scrub will make your skin softer and brighter.

Ingredients:

- One teaspoon of rosewater

- Half a teaspoon of either finely ground almonds or almond flour

Procedure:

1. Wash your face with warm water.

2. Mix together the ingredients.

3. Apply on the face.

4. Wash off with warm water.

Oatmeal Facial Exfoliator

This scrub shall smooth, hydrate and tone your facial skin.

Ingredients:

- One tablespoon of steel-cut oatmeal

- One teaspoon of lemon juice

- Two teaspoons of yogurt

Procedure:

1. Wash your face with warm water.

2. Mix together all the ingredients.

3. Apply the scrub on the face.

4. Allow this to sit on your face for a while so as to serve as a facial mask.

5. Scrub and then rinse with warm water.

Facial Scrub with Honey and Milk

This scrub will moisturize your face.

Ingredients:

- One teaspoon of skim milk if you have oily skin
- One teaspoon of cream milk if you have dry skin
- One teaspoon of milk (2%) for normal skin
- One teaspoon honey
- One tablespoon of ground almonds

Procedure:

1. Combine all the ingredients together
2. Apply on face that has been washed with warm water.
3. Rinse face with warm water again.

Honey Sugar Facial Exfoliator

Ingredients:

- One teaspoon of honey

- Half a teaspoon of brown or cane sugar

Procedure:

1. Wash your face with warm water

2. Combine all ingredients in a bowl

3. Apply on your face

4. Wash your face with warm water.

Chapter 4 – Anti-aging Facial Cleansers

It is necessary to cleanse the skin every day because acne, blackheads and dead skin cells will build up and give you a bad complexion. If you want youthful skin, you need to add a cleanser to your skin care regimen, especially on the face. You can make your own facial cleanser at home if you do not want to use commercial facial washers that have harsh chemicals or if you are on a tight budget.

When you use a facial cleaner, the dullness of your skin will go away and a healthy glow shall replace it. Acne will also be reduced and your skin will appear younger. Make-up will also be removed properly. Here are facial cleansers that will make your skin cleaner and younger.

Refreshing Facial Cleanser

This type of cleanser will help renew your skin because of its Vitamin C content. Milk has been a traditional recipe for cleaning which Cleopatra used. Use this cleanser daily.

Ingredients:

- One ripe tomato

- Two tablespoons of milk

- Two tablespoons of grapefruit, lemon, lime, orange or any citrus fruit

Procedure:

1. Combine all the ingredients in your food processor

2. Wash your face with warm water.

3. Apply the cleanser on your face and then wash with warm water.

Blend the ingredients together in a food processer.

Healing Facial Cleanser

This moisturizer is effective because of its Aloe Vera content which is known to treat a lot of skin conditions. It also has papaya that has healthy enzymes for your skin to remain youthful. It also has honey which serves as an antibacterial and a moisturizer. The yogurt will remove your dead skin cells.

Ingredients:

- One large pealed Aloe Vera leaf
- One small slice papaya that is peeled
- One tablespoon plain yogurt
- One tablespoon honey

Procedure:

1. Combine all the ingredients in your food processor
2. Wash your face with warm water.
3. Apply your cleanser on your face.
4. Rinse your face with warm water.

Notice your skin to feel vibrant and reinvigorated. It will also make it youthful and healthy.

Avocado Facial Cleanser

One of the natural nourishing fruits is avocado. It will make an effective cleanser as it has a lot of vitamins and oils to enhance the skin naturally.

Ingredients:

- One ripe peeled & pitted avocado
- One egg
- Cream
- Two bowls
- Fork

Procedure:

1. Place one-half of your avocado in your bowl and mash this using a fork.
2. Separate the white from the egg and keep the yolk.
3. Put the yolk in the other bowl and beat till it becomes frothy
4. Mix your cream to the egg yolk you beat and combine this with your mashed avocado.
5. Beat this mixture till it becomes smooth.
6. Apply the mixture on your face.
7. Wash your face with warm water afterwards.

Honey & Avocado Facial Cleanser

Ingredients:

- One ripe avocado

- One tablespoon of apple cider vinegar

- One tablespoon of honey

- A small bowl

Procedure:

1. Cut avocado into cubes and place in the bowl.

2. Add your honey and apple cider vinegar and mix till a paste forms.

3. Place the cleanser on your face.

4. Let this sit for ten minutes.

5. Use a damp cloth to take off the cleanser.

6. Wash your face using warm water.

Chapter 5 – Anti-aging Facial Toners

A skincare regimen also needs toning aside from scrubbing and cleansing. Facial toners will make your skin look healthy and clean. You can make facial toners at home if you feel commercial toners are harmful to your skin because of their chemical content. Whatever kind of toner you want to use, be it homemade or commercial, always tone your skin after cleansing and before moisturizing.

Toxins enter the skin and make it look dull and unhealthy. These toxins come from chemicals that you are exposed to every day. Examples are smog, smoke and chemical residues that come from the skin. When you use a facial toner, these toxins are removed and your skin will appear healthier and brighter. You will have less acne, scars and wrinkles.

Toners hydrate your skin and this will make it elastic, smooth, moisturized and younger-looking. When your skin is properly hydrated, it shall minimize aging signs and it will give a good base in preparation to applying cosmetics. There are many toners that give vitamins and other nutrients to the skin so that it remains balanced, healthy and youthful.

Unfiltered Apple Cider Vinegar Toner

This toner is guaranteed to be safe because it does not have preservatives and chemicals that commercial toners have. It is also 100% natural and is inexpensive to make. Unfiltered apple cider vinegar has plenty of nutrients as well as the ingredient called alpha-hydroxy acid which is found in many commercial anti-aging products. This acid balances the pH of the skin, controls oil production and fights skin inflammation and infection.

Ingredients:

- One-third cup of unfiltered ACV

- Three cups of distilled water

- One clean bottle

Procedure:

1. Combine your ingredients.

2. Place the mixture in the bottle.

3. Shake the bottle well.

4. Get a cotton ball and soak it with your ACV toner.

5. Apply your toner on your newly-cleansed face.

You can also make another version of this toner. Instead of the distilled water, use green tea. You can also add a few teaspoons of witch hazel or some drops of tea tree oil so as to kill bacteria that can cause acne. Place your toner in your refrigerator after use.

Green Tea Toner

Ingredients:

- Five green tea bags

- Two cups of vitamin or mineral water

- One clean bowl

- One clean bottle

Procedure:

1. Boil the water.

2. Put your tea bags in the bowl.

3. After the water has boiled, pour this in your bowl.

4. Allow steeping for three minutes.

5. Remove the green tea bags.

6. Place your mixture in your bottle and allow cooling.

7. Soak a cotton ball with your toner and apply on your face.

8. Apply a moisturizer afterwards.

9. Store your bottle in your refrigerator for five days. Discard after five days of use.

The next chapter will tell you how to make homemade moisturizers.

Chapter 6 – Anti-aging Facial Moisturizers

A very important part of caring for your skin is using facial moisturizers. If you moisturize your skin, you can take away its roughness and make it so smooth and soft. The problem with purchasing commercial facial moisturizers is that they can burn a hole in your wallet. They also contain harsh chemicals that will harm your skin, especially if it were sensitive. These include artificial fragrances, dyes and harmful preservatives. This is the reason why such products are very expensive.

If you are on a tight budget, you can make your own facial moisturizers using ingredients in your kitchen. These are just as effective as the commercial ones and they are a lot safer because of the ingredients you will use.

Making your own facial moisturizers to maintain the youthfulness of your skin can be a fun activity to do with your mother, daughter, sister or friends. You will just use natural ingredients such as butter, essential oils, liquids and herbs.

Beeswax Facial Moisturizer

Ingredients:

- Two tablespoons beeswax

- ¾ cup of grape seed or jojoba oil

- Microwave-safe bowl

- Ten drops of your chosen essential oil (orange, lemon or lavender)

- Blender

- Dishwasher detergent

- Once cup of distilled water

- One large glass jar

Procedure:

1. Chop your beeswax in smaller pieces. It is necessary to chop the wax so that it will melt quickly.

2. Put your chopped beeswax in your bowl.

3. Add your grape seed or jojoba oil in the bowl.

4. Place your bowl in your microwave and heat it for 15 seconds in a high setting.

5. Stir the mixture and reheat for another 15 seconds or till you see that the mixture has not thickened. Be careful not to overheat.

6. Place your essential oil in the mixture and stir.

7. Allow the bowl to reach room temperature.

8. Place your blender and its parts, your jar and your spatula in your dishwasher as well as your dishwasher detergent for sterilization.

9. Turn on the dishwasher and then remove its contents once it turns off. In removing the contents, do not touch the rims or its insides so as not contaminate them.

10. Place the mixture in your blender.

11. Add your distilled water.

12. Set the blender at a low speed and check the mixture to see if it thickens to your desired consistency.

13. Have a clean jar ready that can hold not less than two cups of lotion. Make sure to boil the jar so that it will not be contaminated with bacteria.

14. Use a sterilized spatula to take away the mixture from your blender and place this in your sterilized jar.

This is a good moisturizer which you can place on your face and even on your whole body. After six months, throw away the remaining mixture. Make sure to place your moisturizer in a cool place and ensure it is not under direct sunlight. You can place scented water when making this mixture so that you can have the scent you want. Choose the essential oil you desire to achieve a more fragrant smell. Never use tap water when making this moisturizer as this has microbes and chemicals that will deem your homemade facial moisturizer ineffective.

Green Tea Moisturizer

One of the effective moisturizers is green tea as it holds your skin's moisture. Here is a recipe that will make your skin more youthful because it has green tea and Aloe Vera which gets moisture from the surrounding air.

Ingredients:

1. Four tablespoons of grated beeswax

2. Coconut oil

3. Grapeseed oil

4. Measuring cups & spoons

5. One small saucepan

6. Green tea bags or leaves

7. Essential Oils

8. Aloe Vera gel

Procedure:

1. Mix altogether your coconut and grapeseed oil and beeswax inside your saucepan.

2. Melt this over low heat.

3. Place your beeswax and melted oils in a mixing bowl.

4. Allow to cool.

5. Boil green tea and let this steep for five minutes.

6. Use a strainer to remove the green tea remnants.

7. Allow the green tea to cool.

8. Blend your oils with an immersion blender.

9. Pour in your Aloe Vera gel and tea.

10. Blend till it becomes creamy and thick

11. Add your chosen essential oil (a few drops only) during the end of your mixing process

12. Remove the cream and place in a sterilized container using a sterilized spatula.

The eyes will make a person look older because the skin surrounding them is the thinnest of all. It is this skin which ages first so you need to take care of it properly with anti-aging eye creams. Eye creams however are very expensive because of the ingredients they have. Some of these ingredients can also be a bit harmful to sensitive skin. Making your own eye cream at home is more practical and safer.

When making eye creams, gels and serums, you should use natural ingredients. You can add your desired scents like Aloe Vera, cocoa butter or lavender. Here are some recipes you can make to have homemade anti-aging eye creams for your face to look more youthful and radiant.

Anti-Aging Eye Serum

Ingredients:

- Five drops rose essential oil

- Five drops chamomile essential oil

- One ounce jojoba oil

- One clean 1 ounce glass bottle

- Dropper

Procedure:

1. Mix your oils together.

2. Place in your glass bottle.

3. Place a drop of your mixture under your eye and brow bone.

4. Do not place on your eyelids directly.

Wrinkle Anti-Aging Eye Cream

Ingredients:

- Three teaspoons jojoba oil

- Three teaspoons apricot-kernel oil

- One teaspoon beeswax

- One small saucepan

- Five teaspoons rose water

- One-fourth teaspoon of borax

- Five drops carrot-seed essential oil

- Clean glass jar

Procedure:

1. Over low heat, warm jojoba oil, apricot-kernel oil and beeswax in your saucepan.

2. Remove saucepan from your stovetop once heated.

3. Stir the mixture.

4. Warm over low heat the rose water in another saucepan.

5. Add the borax and stir till it dissolves.

6. Remove from the heat and allow this mixture to turn lukewarm.

7. Combine the two blends and stir rapidly.

8. Allow the mixture to cool down to room temperature.

9. Add the carrot-seed essential oil.

10. Place in your glass jar.

11. Apply the eye cream beneath the eyes twice every day before you moisturize.

12. Let this sit for 10 minutes.

13. Remove the cream using a soft cloth

When applying eye creams, use your right ring finger because it is the weakest of all fingers. Again, the skin surrounding the eyes is the most sensitive and thinnest so you need to handle it with much caution and slowness. Do not rub eye cream but pat it softly around your eyes.

Chapter 7 – Anti-aging Facial Masks

The last step in your skin care regimen should be putting on a facial mask. Many people forget this step though because they think it is not at all important. These masks can be expensive when bought at beauty health stores, pharmacies, drugstores and groceries. Beauty spas also charge high when you ask them to put one on you. The good news is you can make a facial mask at home that is just as effective as the ones bought in stores or the ones used in spas.

Honey and Almond Facial Mask

Ingredients:

- One teaspoon of honey
- Six tablespoons evening primrose oil
- Essential oils that are 100% pure
- Two drops mandarin oil
- Two drops orange oil
- Two drops neroli oil
- Two teaspoons of almonds
- Microwavable bowl
- Microwave
- Food processor

Procedure:

1. Collect all the ingredients. You can buy essential oils in beauty shops, health food stores or from the internet.

2. Place your honey in your bowl and put this in your microwave for several seconds.

3. Set your microwave on high power.

4. Combine your evening primrose oil to your warm honey.

5. Mix in your essential oils, mandarin oil, orange oil and neroli oil.

6. Combine altogether the ingredients.

7. Place your almonds in your food processor and grind thoroughly. Make sure no big pieces are left.

8. Place some of your ground almonds in the honey mixture to form a smooth cream.

9. Apply on your skin while it is warm.

10. The mask must be left on your skin for half an hour.

11. Rinse using warm water.

12. Pat-dry your face with a soft cloth

Banana Facial Mask

Bananas can actually be made into a facial mask and it will make your skin look and feel softer and younger. This is a natural way to have a Botox.

Ingredients:

- Medium-sized banana (ripe)

- Cold water

Procedure:

1. Mash your banana to form a smooth paste.

2. Place this on your face.

3. Leave for twenty minutes.

4. Wash with cold water.

You can also mix two tablespoons of honey and one-fourth cup of plain yogurt in your banana before mashing it to make a potent anti-aging facial mask.

Egg, Honey and Orange Juice Mask

Ingredients:

- Two tablespoons of kelp powder

- Egg white of one egg

- Orange juice (natural)

- Small bowl

Procedure:

1. Place your kelp powder in your bowl.

2. Add your egg white into the bowl.

3. Add honey.

4. Add some drops of your natural orange juice.

5. Mix altogether to form a paste.

6. Wash your face using warm water.

7. Apply the mask for 15 minutes.

8. Wash your face with cold water.

This mask is very effective. Kelp is a vegetable found in the sea and it minimizes oil production that causes acne, fights off dark age spots, lessens inflammation and swelling and prevents wrinkles. Wrinkles that are present will be smoothened by kelp.

The egg white will heal and soothe your skin, decrease wrinkles and fine lines, and refine and moisturize the pores. Another good thing about egg white is that it heals burned skin caused by the sun and the wind. It can also tighten loose skin surrounding your face and neck.

The honey helps clean the face because it has antifungal, antiseptic and antibacterial properties that kill bacteria. It will clean and nourish skin that is aging.

The Vitamin C in orange juice will help make the skin look younger. This nutrient helps the skin to make more collagen so it becomes more elastic, smoother and youthful.

Conclusion

Thank you again for purchasing this book!

I hope this book was able to help you to know more about aging skin and what recipes to make to counteract it.

The next step is to go to your kitchen and start making those recipes so that you will look ten years younger after using them.

In addition, please remember to LIKE our Facebook page in order to find other resources and upcoming promotions:

https://www.facebook.com/joypublishing

With sincere thanks,

Charlotte Evans